FROM CLIENT TO CLINIC OWNER

FROM CLIENT TO CLINIC OWNER

Create your wellbeing business from the inside out

Helen Pinnock

From Client to Clinic Owner

Cover art © Lucy Kong, Lucy Kong Creative
www.bidvine.com/pro/lucy-kong-creative

Content Editor: David Pinnock

Interior Design: David Pinnock

Author's note: Out of respect, some names in this book have been changed.

www.wellbeingbusiness–school.com
Facebook: @wellbeingbusinessschool
Instagram: wellbeingbusiness_school

All enquiries: info@helen.pinnock.com

This book is dedicated to my husband David who has always supported me to follow my dreams however crazy they seem. To all my friends and the amazing healers who have crossed my path throughout my wellness journey, none of this would be possible without you all.

"Let yourself be silently drawn by the strange pull of what you really love. It will not lead you astray."

Rumi

CONTENTS

It all starts with you.

CHAPTER ONE

INTRODUCTION

This book is born out of the idea that it is possible to create a business that is heartfelt and successful. But, what does this mean? In my mind, a heartfelt business is run in line with your personal values; all of your interactions should be authentic and genuine.

There is no stress in selling as you fully believe in the service you are offering. You use your personal story to inspire and encourage your clients. A heartfelt business allows you to work with the people you are meant to and provides you with a life you love.

My journey from client to therapist, clinic owner and business coach has spanned twenty years. It has been an interesting path; having to learn the practicalities of running a business combined with a lot of personal self-discovery. I used to look in the mirror and see a shy, self-conscious woman struggling with chronic health issues and no idea what she wanted to do with her life. Now I am a business woman who has created three businesses dedicated to holistic health and wellbeing.

I used to think wellbeing and business were two words and concepts that did not go together; the idea of marketing and charging for my services as a holistic therapist made me feel uncomfortable. This belief caused me a great deal of stress not to mention financial hardship. I was disillusioned and frustrated; I was so desperate to help people with my new-found knowledge, but constantly struggled to find enough clients.

Something had to change……

I turned inwards and began to trust what my intuition was telling me. Over the years I have learned to rely more and more on my intuition. The more you get to know yourself within your business the more powerful your intuition becomes. If I truly listen to my inner voice it very rarely fails me. I quickly realised I had to create a business that fulfilled the whole of me; body, mind and spirit.

The insight and exercises included in the following pages are going to challenge you to gain clarity around who you are here to work with and help you get your message out into the world in a way that fulfils the whole of you. I will share with you the advice I have been given and the lessons I have learned along the way; there are lots of ideas to help you create your unique heartfelt business.

Whilst I do not know what stage you are at in your wellbeing journey, I do know that you are here to help people improve their health and wellbeing.

If I can build a successful practice and clinic then so can you.

At times building a business can feel overwhelming and confusing but, trust me, you have got this far so don't give up, have a little faith in yourself; your future clients will thank you for it.

How to use this book

You can work through this book in chapter order and build your knowledge or dip in at any point to the chapters that feels relevant to you.

Each chapter includes exercises and examples to work through. I suggest you will need to create 2 to 3 hours of distraction free space for yourself to complete each chapter. I would encourage you to hand write the exercises rather than type them into your computer. The act of hand writing is linked to improved creativity, critical thinking and problem solving - all of the skills you will need to create your wellbeing business. I want you to get all those ideas and thoughts you have in your head down on paper because you will be connecting the emotional processing part of your brain with the problem-solving part.

For ease, I am going to use the term wellbeing to cover all the terms for holistic therapies, meditation and yoga.

The world needs
the healing gifts
only you have.

CHAPTER TWO

WHERE IT ALL BEGAN

My journey into discovering the world of wellbeing and complementary therapies started while I was looking for ways to manage my own health issues. I was diagnosed, at the age of 14, with Polycystic Ovary Syndrome (PCOS). PCOS is a lifelong condition that causes irregular and unbelievably heavy periods. It can also make it difficult to conceive, amongst other complications. After ten years of being prescribed a string of heavy painkillers, taking the contraceptive pill (which was meant to alleviate my symptoms) and attending countless dead-end GP and hospital appointments, I grew tired of it all. I felt I had been pushed from pillar to post for far too long and I knew that there had to be another way to control this debilitating condition.

Long before the internet was available for research, I started reading everything I could get my hands on about nutrition and consequently started to experiment with a low carb diet. The self-diagnosed changes that I made helped my periods regain a degree of regularity for the first time in years! It was around this time that I read in a magazine about a woman who got pregnant using homeopathy. At this point I was prepared to give anything a go.

I found a homeopath whose initial consultation left me feeling unsure of myself and my decision to visit her. The room was cold and uninviting, and she did little to explain the process of homeopathy and why she needed the information she was asking me. I felt like her questions were random. For example, "How do I feel when I'm upset?" "What kinds of food do I crave?", etc. Despite this, I intuitively knew this was going to help me. I kept up with the therapy and began to notice improvements in my health.

I was hooked! Wellbeing became my passion. I wanted to know everything. I wanted everyone to know there was a more natural way to take care of your health. The result of this exploration meant that I now have two boys and mostly have my PCOS under control.

I set about training in various therapies, such as Indian head massage, Hopi ear candling and Reiki. But I primarily practised as a reflexologist. All through this period, I could not shake off that first negative impression I had experienced with my homeopathy consultation, at the start of my wellbeing journey.

That first experience of homeopathy taught me that it is not enough to be a talented therapist or teacher. It is equally as important to make clients feel safe in their decision to use complementary therapy, creating a safe and healing environment and taking the time to explain the process.

I loved being a therapist, meeting clients and listening to their stories, so I could help facilitate their healing. But I began to realise that many members of the public wanted complementary health but did not know what treatment was best for them, or where to go to receive it . It was then that I understood   that my time as a therapist was coming to a natural end and it was time to start making complementary therapy more accessible to people in general.

I bought the Wellbeing Clinic in 2004 and set about creating a therapy clinic in line with my ideas, values and beliefs. My intention was to create a more accessible experience for clients and an inspiring environment for therapists.

The past 20 years have been a journey with many ups and downs. I have made mistakes and learnt along the way. The first few years of owning my clinic were particularly challenging I had a vision and no idea how to put it into practice. We were seeing on average only thirty clients a week and had only a handful of therapists working with us.

This small amount was not enough to cover the clinic costs let alone providing a living for me and my family. I realised very quickly that I couldn't keep working the same way and expect a different result. Fast-forward 14 years I now have fourteen therapists on average we deliver between 100 and 130 client sessions a week despite the bad economic client in Britain over the last few years.

This book is an accumulation of things I have learnt and experienced both as a client, therapist and then as a clinic owner and business coach; it is here to help you create the class or practice of your dreams. I believe that creating a wellbeing business that works for you, and fits in with your life and your uniqueness is not about looking outward hoping clients come your way but an inward journey.

When people ask me, "What is the most important thing to learn in order to create a steady stream of clients?", I always give the answer that you need to be prepared to work on yourself, your beliefs, your confidence and your ability to show up and put your ideas into practice. Doing this work is just as important as the normal business tasks such as planning and strategy. If you do not have the right mind set you risk tripping yourself up and getting in your own way.

Bearing this in mind, throughout this book I will be challenging you to look inside of yourself and to work on your beliefs and confidence as well as the practicalities of running a business.

You are here to

make a difference.

CHAPTER THREE

WHAT IS YOUR STORY?

You started your wellbeing business to help people, the objective of your business is to inspire potential clients to take action, to buy your service or attend your class. One way to do this is to share a little of your own story; why you started your wellbeing business. Story telling is a powerful way to connect with your clients. A story is more interesting, more powerful, than a page full of dry facts or bullet points about your therapy/class.

Your story helps people to identify with you and what you have to offer them. We all want to be inspired, especially in the world of wellbeing and health. My Instagram account is littered with inspiring people who have transformed their health naturally. I love watching, reading and listening to their stories because it encourages me to make positive changes in my life.

We buy services and products from people we like, trust and admire. By sharing a little of your story, you are helping potential clients to trust their buying decisions, you are showing them who you are and what you have to offer them.

I have shared a little of my story at the beginning of this book with the hope that you will be inspired to put in the work to create your dream business. Your heartfelt story demonstrates your passion, your excitement for what you do and there is nothing more attractive to a potential client than a therapist/teacher who is passionate about what they do.

Your story is the starting point for everything you want to achieve in your wellbeing business it is the reason you trained in wellbeing and the reason you want to share this message with the world.

Before you panic at the idea of sharing your story with people you do not know, or the idea that you have nothing to share that people would want to read, you can relax. I am not going to ask you to do anything you are not comfortable with.

You may be very comfortable with the idea of sharing your story on your website or talking about it at a networking event, alternatively the idea of sharing anything about yourself may be terrifying.

I want to share with you Cassie's story. Her story inspired me to go along to her paddle board group. I have chronic back pain which means I can struggle to find a sport that suits me. One day I was browsing Facebook and came across a post about a yoga and paddle board teacher called Cassie who ran a group near me, this in itself is a little unusual as I live in a land locked county. I was intrigued and clicked through to her website I read her story it turned out she had been inspired to take up yoga and paddle boarding after suffering from a catastrophic back injury herself.

I was interested, if Cassie could change her life and take up a sport that helped her live her life on her terms then I could give it a try at the very least. I was inspired because I could relate a little to her experiences.

I was sold, I went along and loved it, her enthusiasm for yoga and paddle boarding was infectious. I had found my new sport. By virtue of the fact that she had struggled with her own back pain meant I did not feel the pressure to push myself beyond my limits, so I was able to relax and enjoy myself.

This is just one example of how I have been inspired by someone's story. I am sure you can think of your own examples.

Your own story about why you became a therapist, meditation or yoga teacher is important there are people in your area who want and need a little inspiration, encouragement or motivation. Your story may be just what they need.

Before you say but I don't have a story. Yes, you do, we all have a story. It may not seem dramatic or life changing to you, but every one of us has had successes and failures and all of our lives are meaningful.

As I have already mentioned I do not want you to share anything about yourself you are not comfortable with. I believe there are some details of all our lives, that should be kept for friends, family or the therapy room.

The exercise below will help you not only write your story but also help you explore where your own boundaries lie. As in life, it is important to have clear boundaries within your business. Boundaries help us protect our own emotional and physical energy. They help us to stay focused and keep us living in line with our values. Writing down your story will help you work out where these boundaries lie for you.

Over the years my boundaries have changed and I am much happier to share more about myself today than I was when I first started as a reflexologist.

TAKE ACTION

___

Write your story

Yes, this may be challenging but I would really encourage you to give it a go. Write as though you are talking to a friend, this will help you to keep it simple, friendly and authentic, resist the urge to use long fancy words. Keep it simple and unfiltered:

- Beginning – what was your challenge, what did you overcome?
- Middle – what decisions or actions did you take to make a change in your life?
- End – what was the result of your decisions or actions?

There is no right or wrong. It can be very hard to write about yourself but we all have to start somewhere. Once you have written something down, put it to one side and leave it for a while. When you come back to it I want you to ask yourself:

- With which bits of this am I happy sharing with the world?
- Is this story going to be inspiring to my potential clients?
- By reading my story will they see that they can also make positive changes in their lives?

If you struggle with this ask a trusted friend to read it and ask their opinion.

Having answered these questions, you may want to rewrite or refine your story before sharing it with potential clients.

If, once you have written your story, you are still not comfortable with sharing I want you to know that this is ok. This process will have helped you to clarify your 'WHY' and what it is that motivated you to choose wellbeing as a career path. This information will be useful to you as you move through the book; it will help you to write your mission statement, identify your ideal client and give you the clarity you will need to keep moving forward, especially when business feels a little tough.

Live a life that

matters to you.

CHAPTER FOUR

CREATE A MISSION STATEMENT FOR YOUR LIFE AND BUSINESS?

Congratulations you have trained in your chosen wellbeing therapy/class, you are excited to get going to treat and help as many people as possible. However, I believe there are some more steps to take before you begin advertising and marketing your services – doing the normal business stuff.

In the previous chapter, you have told your story and you have found your 'WHY'. Now you need to develop an even deeper understanding about your purpose and mission. What is at the heart of your wellbeing business? What do you value - what is your wellbeing mission? Why are you doing it and what do you stand for?

You may think mission statements are an out-dated concept or just for companies that have employees. This is not the case; creating a personal mission statement for yourself will help you to move your wellbeing business in a direction that fits with your personal beliefs and values. It will help you achieve your goals not just in your business but in your personal life as well. It will help you build an authentic brand that demonstrates your uniqueness.

Below is an example of a wellbeing business mission statement. Even though they are often only a single sentence you get an immediate sense of what their business stand for, what it is that matters to them.

"My get-the-glow philosophy is all about enjoying what makes you feel happy and healthy." Madeline Shaw

Until I discovered wellbeing I drifted from job to job. I had a vague notion that I wanted to help people in some way but had not found a job that met this need. Although I was earning a living, I felt unsatisfied. At the same time, I was struggling with my own health and unhappy with the advice and treatment I was receiving. No one seemed to be taking me seriously; the medication I was being offered was not helping my hormones, in reality, they were making them worse. I felt as though I had lost control of what was happening to my body. I felt invisible, a number in a big machine.

When I discovered complementary therapy as a way to help my own health it did not just help me regulate my cycle and conceive my children it also helped me to regain my confidence and sense of self. I had found what I wanted to do with my life; I became passionate about helping women regain control of their bodies and came up with a list of statements that said what I wanted to do:

- I wanted to help women regulate their own bodies naturally.

- I wanted to create a wellbeing business I felt passionate about - something I could put my heart and soul into.

- I wanted to help women to feel seen and heard.

- I wanted to help women feel they had the power to make decisions about their own health.

Most people have a broad sense of what they stand for in their wellbeing business however, a lot of people struggle to get specific with their mission. It does require you to do some introspection. A good place to start is to work out what your personal values are, what it is you value most.

For example, if you are someone who values honesty, connection and learning then these three values should become part of everything you do in your wellbeing business; from how you interact with clients, to how you write your website.

When I do this exercise with my coaching clients it often takes them some time to get comfortable with it. So be gentle with yourself and make sure you allow yourself the space and time to contemplate the answers.

I want you to think deeply when doing this exercise - you will have many values that you live your life by. I want you to question whether they are really yours or are they the values society wants you to have? As we go through life we take on board the values of our parents, teachers and friends. This exercise is about getting to the heart of what really matters to you.

Bearing this is mind, please remember there is no right or wrong answer to this, your values are your own, they are what makes you who you are.

TAKE ACTION

How to work out your core values

This exercise consists of three stages.

- Contemplating

- Choosing

- Committing

Stage 1: Contemplating

I want you to start by writing a list of values that matter to you. I have included a few suggestions to get your started write everything you can think of. Do not limit or filter yourself. We will narrow it down as we go.

Examples:

- Truth

- Learning

- Connection

- Authenticity

- Family

- Intimacy

- Kindness

- Empowerment

- Openness

- Passion

- Service

- Health

- Wellbeing

- Creativity

- Empathy

- Support

- Love

- Honesty

Stage 2: Choosing

From the list, you compiled I want you to choose seven values and then put them in order of importance the most important one at the top. Once you have done this take each of the values and complete the following phrase.

"What does the word _____ mean to me?"

Under each phrase write an answer.

Stage 3: Committing

Now you have your seven values and what they mean to you, I want you to narrow it down even more. Which three of your seven values could you not live without? Take as much times as you need to work this out.

Now you have your three value statements I want you to notice if there are any common themes among them. Now have a go at writing a value statement that includes the three values you have identified.

Here is an example of a value statement from Whole Foods – "The world's leading organic and natural grocer.":

"With great courage, integrity and love—we embrace our responsibility to co-create a world where each of us, our communities, and our planet can flourish, all the while, celebrating the sheer love and joy of food."

Whole Foods

Narrowing your values down to just three can be very challenging so go easy on yourself. If you need a break whilst doing this then take it. One of my coaching clients gave herself an entire week to do this. Yes, it took time but she gained a huge amount of insight and clarity around who she is and how she wanted her mindfulness business to look. Using her personal values, she was able to write a personal mission statement that worked for her business. Keeping this statement in mind she re-wrote her website and changed her style of writing to reflect what was important to her.

The process of working out what mattered to her gave her the courage to speak her true voice and not hide behind what she thought she should say. The result was that her passion, integrity and knowledge came through. She was able to set goals for her business that were in line with what she valued. The result was that she attracted; she had more clients that resonated with her own beliefs. Her business filled up and her work became more fulfilling. Fundamentally, her business was not in conflict with her personal values.

Having completed this task, you should now have a clearer idea about what your personal values are which will enable you to create your wellbeing business your way. Every decision you make, every goal you set, will be in line with these values.

This means you can bring your full authentic self to your wellbeing business. By working in line with our values we are more committed to our own success we have more energy, creativity, enthusiasm and most importantly less stress because we fully believe in what we are doing.

Set yourself goals
that make your
heart sing

CHAPTER FIVE

SET MEANINGFUL GOALS THAT MAKE YOUR HEART SING

Goal: "The object of a person's ambition or effort; an aim or desired result."

Dictionary Definition

Any wellbeing business owner, no matter where they are in their business life, needs to create goals for their business:

- Mindful goals help you to achieve your wellbeing mission.

- Goals keep your business, therapy and classes moving forward.

- Well thought out meaningful goals in line with your personal values should provide you with the motivation to carry them out.

- Your clients have goals for their health and wellbeing. By setting goals for yourself you are encouraging them to continue working on theirs.

- A measurable goal will show you when you have been successful, it will also show you when you need to stop, revaluate and change direction.

That being said, I know many of my coaching clients associate the idea of goal setting with stress and fear. They worry about not being able to achieve the goals they set themselves. In this chapter I want to show you different ways you can mindfully set goals that are in line with your unique mission.

We will look at tools to help you set goals, such as vision boards, list making and the SMART acronym. Once you have used these I want you to take it further and look at how achieving these goals will make you feel.

Vision Boards

A vision board is a visual representation of your dreams and goals. Vision boards are a popular, fun and creative tool to help you envision how you want your business to look.

You can create either a tangible board in your office space or a virtual board on your computer. Pinterest is an excellent resource to help you with this.

Using pictures and images to represent your goals can help you strengthen and get in touch with your emotions, our minds react strongly to visual stimulation.

Whilst creating your board it is important to think, not just about the material and physical goals you want to achieve, but also, how you will feel upon achieving them.

Personally, I prefer a tangible vision board that hangs above my desk; something that I can look at often. I don't find this so easy when it is on my computer. The ability to be able to look at your vision board often stimulates your creativity and encourages your subconscious brain.

TAKE ACTION

Now it is time to create your own vision board however, before you do, you need to have an idea of what your goals are; the purpose of the vision board is to help you develop your goals and achieve them.

- The following process will help:
- Make a list of your goals and ambitions for the next 12 months let yourself dream.
- If you are going to make a physical board collect some old magazines with beautiful

pictures. If you don't have enough ask your friends.

- Now make time, preferably a couple of hours, to cut out pictures that represent these goals. Use pictures that speak to you. If you are making an online board the same applies collect the images that you are attracted to.

- Now make your board. Glue, stick, pin in a way that is pleasing to you.

- Now you have your board it is important to realise that goals are not just about material gain they are also about how you want to feel. So, take some sticky notes and write a feeling word for every one of your images. I suggest that you use some of these feeling words on your board; words such as joy, freedom, healthy, strong, and powerful.

- Do not worry about your goals and vision board being set in stone you can keep going back to your vision board as often as necessary.

If vision boards don't feel the right way to create and develop your goals, you can of course just write them down in a list; as long as you can turn these goals into achievable actions. Try the exercise below; you can always develop the list into a vision board at a later date.

TAKE ACTION

Write a list of goals for the coming 12 months. Here are some of my suggestions:

- 5 more people in my class.
- To train in a certain modality.
- Make a living out of your chosen therapy.
- Earn x amount of money a month.
- Own a yoga studio.
- Own a therapy centre.

Once you have your list you need to take it one step further, as with the vision board, you need to know how you would feel if you achieved these goals. Next to each goal write an emotion.

Working out how you want to feel when you achieve your goal will help to motivate you to get to where you want to be.

For the last few years I have successfully used both these methods to create goals for my wellbeing business that resonate with how I want to feel. The more you use these methods the easier it becomes.

Whenever I have tried to work towards goals that do not resonate with the way I want to feel, or reflect my personal values I have created untold stress for myself. If you are relentless in the pursuit of goals, without stopping to check in with yourself and your intuition, you can destroy your confidence and self-esteem. A misplaced goal can become a tool to create guilt and feelings of failure.

By now you should have your goals and an idea of how you want to feel when you have achieved them. The next step is to turn your goals into reality, but bear in mind some of them may just not be achievable in 12 months. Let us now look at the SMART acronym.

SMART

This acronym consists of the five elements Specific, Measurable, Achievable, Relevant and Time Based. This is a simple tool that is used by many businesses to turn vague goals into an actionable plan.

- **S**pecific (refine your goal to a simple statement).

- **M**easurable (how are you going to define when you have achieved your goal?).

- **A**chievable (is the goal you have set yourself achievable?).

- **R**esources (do you have what you need to achieve your goal? i.e. finances, skills).

- **T**ime Based (does the goal have to be achieved in a certain time?).

TAKE ACTION

Using the SMART acronym, test each of your goals. For example, you may be a Reiki practitioner and you would like to increase your practice numbers; this is your broad goal.

- **S**pecific (I will acquire four new clients for my Reiki business)

- **M**easurable (I will measure my progress by how many new clients I see, while still seeing my current clients.)

- **A**chievable (I will create a social media marketing campaign and attend a local networking event.)

- **R**esources (I need to make time to attend to my marketing on my computer and the fee to attend the networking event.

- **T**ime Based (I will have four new clients within six weeks.)

Meditation and visualisation

I would not claim to meditate on a regular basis or fully understand all the benefits of visualisation. However, they are methods I like to use from time to help me bring clarity to my goals; visualization helps me reach the intended results.

The practice of meditating helps me cut out all the unnecessary and overwhelming clutter of my mind. Your mind is hugely powerful, taking the time to tap into its power and wisdom can bring amazing benefits.

TAKE ACTION

———

If the idea of visualisation is new to you, take one of the goals that you have run through the SMART acronym, now imagine you have completed this goal. Create a visual picture in your mind's eye; how does it sound, smell, look, taste - the more detail you can give your image the better. Now send this image all the positive energy and intention you can, envisage a time and date you would like to achieve this goal in the real world. Take the time to think about any steps you would need to take to make this happen and visualise them happening.

When you feel as though you have completed this take the time to ground yourself and write down everything you have worked with. Next take the necessary steps to achieve your goal. A small action every day will move you to where you want to be. When I have done this in practice, I have found it to be very powerful. I become acutely aware of opportunities and people that can help me achieve my goal.

Resistance to goal setting

Some of you might still be feeling some resistance to the idea of setting goals for yourself. Let us look at why this might be.

Maybe you are lacking a little self-belief in your ideas. If this is what you are feeling I suggest you go back to chapter 4 and work a little more on your mission statement. Your mission statement will help you gain the clarity and self-belief in your idea. It will help you feel confident setting goals in line with your values.

In my experience, some wellbeing business owners actually have a fear they might achieve their goals and become successful. I am aware this one might sound a little strange but I am sure some of you can resonate with this.

Another reason therapists struggle to set meaningful goals is a sense of unworthiness. They feel that they do not deserve to achieve their goals, dreams or desires.

If you recognise this in yourself it deserves some attention. Whilst most of us feel like this sometimes, if it is stopping you creating a successful business then it is a problem. When you do not really believe that you deserve success, you will be projecting a sense of unworthiness out to the world and your clients.

Ask yourself. "Are your feelings of unworthiness mixed up with an idea that you are not good enough or a misplaced idea about perfection?" The need for everything to be perfect can paralyse us in to doing nothing at all. If your ideas need to be perfect all the time it can create a feeling of overwhelm, if you cannot start your goals until the time is right you may never start, if a goal is not perfect you may fail. These negative thoughts and emotions can play havoc with your goal setting.

Unworthiness is sneaky, it comes in many different guises

- Imposter syndrome - I am making a living. Who am I to work with or teach people about their health and wellbeing?

- I am not qualified enough, I have not been qualified long enough.

- No one will like my blog or newsletter. Who do I think I am to write a blog?

I am sure you can add a couple of your own negative self-beliefs to the list. I think it is important to realise that every single person with whom I have worked has faced at least one these doubts from time to time.

The first step to working with these negative beliefs is acknowledging to yourself that you struggle in this area and then noticing if these beliefs are stopping you achieving your goals or even setting them in the first place.

"You are worthy of your desires"

Recognise this? Let us flip these beliefs around.

Assume you had a client who was struggling with these negative beliefs. I am sure you would not teach or facilitate healing in your clients by suggesting that they are not worthy of feeling well or having full health. So, quite simply, why would you think differently for yourself?

I am a great believer in affirmations to help change negative beliefs. When you use a positive affirmation over and over again you are telling your brain that this message is important to you and your brain will start to look for ways to help you achieve this goal. Secondly a positive affirmation is working on a higher level than what you currently believe to be true, by repeating the affirmation over and over you are helping your brain to work on a higher level. Try to repeat your affirmation for at least a month it takes time - for change to occur:

- I am worthy of my desires

- I deserve a life full of achievement, love and success

- I am worthy of my dreams

Pick an affirmation that resonates with you then write it in a place where you will see it. On your phone, on your mirror, whatever it takes and wherever you look the most.

If you are still struggling then let me tell you are worthy of your desires. I believe in you and your dreams. If your goals bring you positive emotions, you will find an ease and joy in the hard work it takes to achieve them.

Note of caution:

A goal is just that. Sometimes we might be called to change direction from what we felt was the right decision at the time. By using the tools, you have learned in this chapter. The importance of your feelings when setting goals and the SMART acronym you will have created ways to measure whether your goals are working for you. It is ok to change direction, even mid-way through your goal, as I have done in the past.

In 2016, I was convinced that the time had come to sell the therapy business I had spent the past 12 years building up. I thought I had achieved all the goals that I had set myself. I felt as though I had given everything I had to the business and it was time to move on. I have a constant desire to feel creatively inspired and I thought this was no longer happening. So, I set the wheels in motion to sell the business, I even told my employees.

But then it all started to feel wrong. I used the SMART acronym to test my goals. I realised I had made a mistake and selling was not going to give me the feelings I wanted, I was not done with the business or the people or wellbeing. I called a stop to the sale, made the changes I needed to make, and felt the way I wanted to feel all along.

I hope this chapter has shown you that goal setting does not need to be overwhelming or overly rigid. By breaking goal setting down into manageable tasks you can create a plan for your success.

What is it all about – what are you here to do?

CHAPTER SIX

WHO IS YOUR IDEAL CLIENT?

Let us reflect a bit. You have told your story, gained clarity about your mission, set some goals and got

to the heart and soul of who you are and what it is you want to achieve. Now you have to work out who your clients are; who you are meant to be teaching and treating, who it is you are trying to get your message in front of.

There are a lot of wellbeing businesses; the vast majority of them offering amazing services. In my local area, there are three complementary health clinics and a lot of independent therapists. So, how do clients choose the one with whom they want to spend their hard-earned money?

In this chapter, we will look at how clients make buying decisions and how, by narrowing down the clients you market to, you can make your wellbeing business stand out in a crowded market place. I want you to think of the last time you paid for a yoga class or chose a therapist. Why were you drawn to them? Is it because it felt like they were speaking to you personally?

Let me give you an example; you are looking for a yoga class but you been diagnosed with fibromyalgia. You know yoga would help but so many of the pictures you see online are of young flexible women with washboard stomachs. So, you feel intimidated, even a bit scared, to go along to the class in case you cannot do any of the exercises or you are worried that other women might stare at you.

Then one night as you are browsing your social media accounts on the internet, a post pops up talking about a yoga class that is designed to help people who suffer with fibromyalgia. Alongside the post there is a picture of a group of happy smiling people who look like you. You are interested and click through to the website and read a little about the yoga teacher who runs the class it turns out she was diagnosed with fibromyalgia 5 years ago. She turned to yoga and has never looked back. It feels as though this yoga teacher has spoken to you directly so you find the nearest class she has and book your place.

In the same area as this first yoga class there is another teacher who is also very good at helping people who suffer with fibromyalgia but she has not talked about this in any of her marketing for fear of putting off clients with other wellbeing issues. Unfortunately, because she is not narrowing down who she is talking to, her marketing is very general; there is nothing to identify her classes as different from anyone else's. Consequently, the second yoga teacher is struggling to fill her classes.

The example above demonstrates why narrowing down who you market to works; it allows you to work with the clients you are best placed to serve.

Before we look at how to help you identify who are your idea clients, let us address the belief that you are here to work with everyone. I believe everyone who starts in business struggles with the idea that they should narrow their target market. This is for a number of reasons, odds on you feel that your chosen therapy or class can help everyone and you are scared to narrow your market in case you miss a potential client. I completely understand these fears however, by now I hope you are beginning to realise you are not here to personally help everyone.

Trying to market to everyone is a recipe for disaster. A 20-year-old woman, who lives in the city, will not receive or hear information in the same way as a 49-year-old woman with 2 children, full-time job and an aging parent she looks after. If we do not get specific about who our ideal clients are we risk blending into the crowd and talking to no one.

Blanket marketing does not work. No matter who your service or class is suitable for. Just as in life, you are not going to suit everyone, and not everyone is going to understand, value or like what you do. By attempting to talk to everyone, you risk becoming white noise and disappearing into all the other information your customers are being bombarded with every day. You will be physically and emotionally drained trying to appeal to everyone.

Now that you appreciate why you should not try to appeal to everyone, I want you to work out who you are supposed to be working with. The following exercise will help you do this.

TAKE ACTION

———

How to create your ideal client

I want you to hold an individual in your mind's eye who you can relate to, if you have a photograph of this person even better. It could be a person you have treated in your therapy room or have in your class already. This individual is someone you feel you are doing, or have done, some good work with. Do not panic if you do not have any clients or classes yet, imagine a friend, colleague or family member, someone who fits your idea of an ideal client.

(Note to remember: You can do this exercise as many times as you like until you get the right fit.)

Next, I want you to answer the following questions as fully as you can imagining they are your ideal client. It may seem a bit odd but go with it. Please do not worry if you can not find the exact information to these questions just take an educated guess. The idea is to get a rounded picture of your ideal client.

Are they......

- male or female?
- married, a partner or single?

Do they........

- have children and if so how many and what age are they?
- work what kind of job do they do they work full time/part time?

- have any disposable income?

- communicate through e-mail or text?

What.........

- kind of car do they drive?

- age are they?

- are their favourite book, magazine, blogs?

- are their interests.

- size house do they live in do they rent or own?

- social media sites do they use?

Where...........

- do they live?

- do they buy their groceries?

- do they shop for clothes?

- do they socialise?

- do they take holidays?

How.............

- do they take care of their health/their families health?

After completing the above task, you should have a very good idea of who your ideal client is. I recognise this can be a difficult task for some people. They struggle with the idea of narrowing down so specifically who they are going to market to. However, I would encourage you to try.

If my coaching clients get stuck and overwhelmed with this task I suggest they stand in front of a mirror and take a good long look at themselves often our ideal client is the person looking back at us. It stands to reason that for many of us we are best suited to working with clients who are like us; those clients who have had similar experiences to us, those clients who can relate to our story. If your ideal client is someone just like you do not be tempted to skip the above task; doing it will still help you gain insight about your marketing and how you receive information.

What to do with the information you now have?

You should now have a wealth of information about who your ideal client is - so it is time to use it. The information you have gathered will help you tailor your marketing to speak directly to your potential clients. Below are some of the ways in which you will use your ideal client profile.

- Every time you write copy for your social media, leaflet or website hold your ideal client in your mind. A little tip I use is to write copy as though I am writing this person an e-mail.

- Your ideal client will help you to decide where to work from and when. If your ideal client is a 20-year-old female you may decide to run classes from a city centre either at lunch time or after work. If your ideal clients are mums with young school age children you may decide to time your therapy sessions within school hours at a therapy centre within the suburbs.

- Where you place your advertising will depend on where your ideal clients look, read and socialize.

- How much disposable income your ideal client has will affect how you price your services.

Stepping into your client's shoes allows you to empathize with them and their situation. It allows you to offer treatments and classes that make them feel heard, seen and understood. After all, is this not something that we all want.

Give yourself
permission to
dream and be
inspired.

CHAPTER SEVEN

DREAM BIG AND DO YOUR RESEARCH

Market research may not seem like the most exciting subject however, it can make a big difference to the success of your wellbeing business.

I would really encourage you to spend some time doing your research. In this chapter, we will discuss the reasons why you should do your market research as well as why many wellbeing businesses skip this part of their planning process. Lastly, we will cover how to do the research to get the results you need to be successful.

In the previous chapters, you have already spent time investigating who is your ideal client is. This however, is not the only thing you should research. Market research is useful for many areas of your business from testing out your business idea to testing your business name and logo, other areas include.

- The appearance and ease of use of your website

- Are the clients you think you want to work with in the area you want to work

- Are your ideal clients available to attend appointments or classes at the times you are free to work?

- The quality of your work

- A new class or therapy

- To support a business plan

- How to price your therapy or class

TAKE ACTION

I would like you to consider this example to provide a better understanding of why you need to do your research. You have recently qualified as a meditation teacher. You have a passion for helping stressed out millennials. You have been offered a room in a therapy centre in the middle of the city but the space is only available between midday and 1pm. Whilst your intuition is telling you that you can get enough clients to come to your meditation class you decide to do some research to check whether this is true or not.

Spend some time thinking about the kind of research you would need to do to get the answers as to whether it is a good idea to run a lunch time meditation class in the centre of a city.

- You could do a quick visual check to see how many businesses are within 10 minutes' walk of the therapy centre. This would give you an indicator of many people would be available to come to your class.

- Is there anyone else offering lunch time meditation classes? If there is someone else offering meditation within the same area do not let that put you off it shows there is a need.

- If there are cafés local to the therapy centre you could ask what the average age of their clients are and whether they would be happy to let you leave some leaflets about the class.

- You could telephone a couple of the local business and ask on average how long their employees take for lunch and at what time.

This may be an imaginary exercise but depending on the result of the research you conduct you would then decide whether to run the class at lunch time in the city or change the venue and time to something more suitable to the needs of your future clients. You may decide you can run the class but make it 45 min rather than 60 min to allow people to return to work.

Imaginary exercise or not, this does show a little research can give you a wealth of information.

As a small business owner, it has never been easier to do research; you can find a lot out by simply spending an hour on your computer.

- The internet is a great place to research competitors who are offering similar services to you.

- Mail chimp and Survey Monkey are great platforms to create online questionnaires and polls. There are many video tutorials to show you how to do this.

- Research can be as simple as having conversations with your existing clients.

- Standing on your local high street is another option however, it is more expensive and challenging, requiring permits and a huge amount of time.

- Social media is a great way to do research. Find a Facebook group that you resonate with and ask questions within the group.

Learning the value of market research

My first business coach gave me a lot of motivation to keep going to create the wellbeing business I dreamt of however, it was my second business coach taught me the value of doing research and the benefits of paying attention to the finer details.

After our first coaching session, he wanted me to research all the competition I had in my local area to the Wellbeing Clinic. At first, I was very resistant to the idea, I was convinced I already knew who my competition was and felt it was an unnecessary use of my time. After all, the reason, I was coming to him was to help me get more clients, I could not see how it would help.

However, he was determined I should do the research, so I did and was surprised by the results. I actually had a lot more competition than I realised; it turned out there were over thirty reflexologists within a 5-mile radius of my own practice and numerous other therapists I was equally unaware of as well as another therapy clinic opening.

Whilst my intuition had told me that I had a lot of competition it had not provided me with the detail I needed. The result of doing this research showed me not just how much competition I had but why I needed to specialise and stop trying to blanket market to everyone. It had shown my why I needed to look at all of the ways I could make my practice stand out from others.

I now use market research to check my intuition is right, by paying attention to the fine details of the research I am able to round out my ideas, fill in the details and turn them into reality.

I suggest you to not only do research when you first start your wellbeing business but throughout your wellbeing career. In my local area two new therapy clinics have opened up in the last 10 years more therapists and teachers are being trained every day. It is important you keep an eye on what is going on. How your clients' needs are changing. For example, within the yoga industry there are new trends emerging every day; clients have the opportunity to try everything from Ariel yoga to yoga in a brewery.

To stay relevant, you need to ensure you know what is going on in your industry and your local area.

TAKE ACTION

———

I challenge you to do some research that will benefit your business whether it is finding out how many other therapists do the same therapy as you within a 5-mile radius or finding out if your dream of opening a yoga studio in your local town is viable.

Know your worth,
do not settle for
anything less.

CHAPTER EIGHT

HOW MUCH SHOULD YOU CHARGE?

Working out what price to charge for your therapy or class is a huge topic. Previously you have worked out who your ideal client is, now we need to match your pricing with your ideal client. The price you settle on is not just about how much money you make; potential clients will make judgments about you and your business based on the price you charge.

Many wellbeing businesses consistently undercharge. We will examine why this is and what to do about it. By the end of this chapter you will understand how to price your business in a way that you feel comfortable with.

The Basics

Before you can decide on a price for your therapy or class you need to know how much it costs you to deliver this class or treatment. This may seem obvious but many people forget to work it out. You need to work out your expenses; how much does it cost you to treat an individual or teach a class. Don't forget to include all expenses for example;

- Hire of room

- Advertising

- Travel

- Equipment

- Insurance

- Training

- Your time

- Website

- Washing towels

Now you have worked out your basic expenses let us look at how pricing should be part of your marketing strategy. Below is an exercise that will demonstrate how your clients will make decisions about you based purely on price. As you work through this I want you to think about how you make buying decisions based on price.

TAKE ACTION

———

I want you to imagine you are going to get a Swedish massage in a city you have never visited before. You want to book a Swedish massage, but the only information you have is the name of the business and their price.

- Wellbeing Rooms: cost £100

- The Retreat Centre   cost £15

- Natural Therapy Clinic   cost £45

How do you decide which massage will suit you? Ok, so this exercise may seem a little simplistic but let me suggest some possible thoughts you had.

The cost of the Wellbeing Rooms is the most expensive and may well be out of your price range but you may well have thought. "They must be good if they can charge that much." At the other end of the scale The Retreat Centre is very cheap, you may have thought. "They can't be very good if that is all they are charging." Bearing that in mind you may decide to go with the Natural Therapy Clinic.

Your thought process may have been entirely different to mine; there is no right or wrong. The point is to get you to think about how you make buying decisions and to realise your clients will be doing the same.

Doing this exercise should demonstrate to you why the price you charge is part of your marketing mix. We all make judgments about a product or service based on the price whether it is a massage or a cup of coffee.

Now you have considered how your clients view pricing we need to look at how your beliefs effect the way you price your therapy or class, particularly undercharging as this is the area with which most wellbeing businesses struggle.

Why do you undercharge for your therapy or class?

There are many reasons wellbeing businesses undercharge. As we have shown earlier in the chapter it may just be down to a lack of knowledge around the importance of price setting or our personal beliefs around money.

When we are new to business we often have a belief that charging less than our competitors, will bring more customers our way. The reality is this very rarely happens. Most clients are not influenced by a few pounds decrease in price. Loyalty, trust, connection and your skills as a teacher-therapist are more important to a client than saving a few pounds.

You may have the belief that discounting your services will make you more available to clients on a lower income. Like it or not, what you are offering is a lifestyle service, if people do not have the money a small discount is unlikely to make a difference to whether they can afford to use your services. However, this does not mean you cannot give back to the community I know therapists who offer a morning a month for a charity free of charge or give a gift voucher for a raffle prizes.

Many newly qualified therapists/teachers struggle to charge a reasonable price. They measure themselves against other therapists/teachers who have more experience. Let us look at it another way. Whilst experience counts for a lot, it is easy to under value your training and skills. As a newly qualified therapist, your skills will be fresh and up to date. You took the time and dedication to train in your chosen therapy, therefore, you deserve to be valued for the work you have put in.

However, it is not just new therapists who struggle to charge what they are worth. I have worked with many therapists who have been in business 10 years plus and then begin to struggle. They see other therapists surpassing them and do not understand why, as Kate's story demonstrates.

A few years ago, I met an amazing acupuncturist called Kate who had an amazing depth of experience. Kate had worked with many clients and had done some incredible work for over ten years. However, in the last three years she was becoming discouraged as her practice was only half full. Less experienced acupuncturists were full and she was struggling to see why, at this point Kate was considering giving up.

After talking to her for a little while I began to feel that something just did not add up. I asked Kate what she was charging for each treatment. It turned out her treatments were cheaper than her less experienced colleagues. Delving a little deeper, it transpired that Kate's clients were even volunteering to pay Kate more money. We talked a little about why she was charging so little for her classes when she had so much experience and then worked a little around her beliefs about money. I suggested that she tried raising her prices to reflect her level of experience.

After some initial concerns, she did this. The result: within three months Kate's practice was full and she had a waiting list.

Kate's pricing and marketing now matched her level of experience, her clients were able to feel and see the congruity which ultimately made them feel safe in her knowledge and ability.

Over the years Kate had become fearful of showing her true self, and her incredible abilities. As a teacher and healer, Kate was keeping herself small and people were missing out on her ability to increase their wellbeing.

I know that some wellbeing business struggle with the idea of charging at all for services that help people:

- Earning money makes me less spiritual

- Money is evil, corrupt and makes me greedy

- If I have too much money other people will go without

Take a moment to think of someone who you respect, who has the values you consider important, someone who has a lot of money. Would they be any different if their finances were different?

I am sure you became a therapist or teacher with the desire to share an abundance of wellbeing and good health with your clients. You can have a healthy relationship with money; providing the best that you can to the clients you are supposed to serve, you are creating abundance, security and freedom for them, and yourself.

I do not believe in the view that there is a scarcity of abundance, love, money, whatever you like to call it. Do not keep yourself small through fear of being seen. Value yourself as you would want others to see you. Value your training and your gifts.

I have tried to show you some of the reasons why setting a price can be difficult. Let us look at how to set your price. There are many proven formulas to setting your price however, do not over complicate it.

Pricing strategy

You should by now have worked out how much it costs to deliver your therapy-class as well as seeing how pricing affects client's perceptions about the value of your service based on price.

Before making a final decision about what price to charge you need to make yourself aware of what your competitors are charging.

TAKE ACTION

———

You will need a computer to do this task I want you to research your competitors within a 5-mile radius of where you work. Make a list of your competitors and the price they charge. (Do not get stuck in the detail, a feel for the price will suffice).

With this list, you can decide where you want to position yourself. An expensive price suggests a premium service, whilst a cheap price suggests a lower level of service.

Although I have been in business for a long time I still review our clinic prices every year to help keep us in line with the local market. I like the clinic to be priced slightly higher than the local average. I feel this reflects the values of the clinic; we value our customer service and therapists offer a high level of treatment and service. We hold our clients at the heart of every decision we make.

Throughout this chapter we have looked how pricing needs to be part of your marketing mix. How pricing can affect how your clients view you and value your service. The importance of being aware of our own money beliefs and what our competitors are charging. Although ultimately only you can decide what to charge for your therapy/class, you should now have the tools to make an informed decision in line with your beliefs and values - a price that allows you to create abundance for yourself and the best service you can provide.

You are making a

difference.

CHAPTER NINE

GETTING YOUR MESSAGE OUT INTO THE WORLD

You have created your wellbeing business now it is time to promote it – to market it. Not everybody understands the concept of selling and marketing so let us consider why it is necessary. It is not about selling to people what they do not need but showcasing the wellbeing services you have to offer. You need to get your message in front of your ideal clients in a way that resonates with you as well as them. You have to let people know about the wellbeing services you are offering. You need to make it easy for them to find you and communicate in a way that is relevant to your ideal clients. You need to make it easy for them to love and trust you, show them what you have to offer and the value you can bring to their health and wellbeing.

Basically, you need to:

- Tell people who you are and what you have to offer.

- Once you have their attention you have to persuade them to take action to buy your wellbeing services rather than your competitors.

- Provide your wellbeing therapy/class then follow up with amazing customer service and request a referral or testimonial.

I find it helpful to think of my marketing as a continuous loop.

There are many marketing methods to choose from, but how do you choose? Hopefully, now you will have done your market research, identified who your ideal client is, where they live and work and how they gather information. This is the first step in deciding how to use your marketing resources.

Here are two examples for different ideal clients.

- Your ideal client is a thirty something female who gathers all her information from social media, recommendations from friends and searching the internet.

- Your ideal client may be a fifty something female who gathers her information from local magazines, attending talks and reading informative blog posts.

As you can see, they gather their information differently, so it makes sense to direct your marketing efforts in a way that will work for your ideal client.

Whilst a website and social media are vital tools for any modern wellbeing business, there are many other marketing methods that will help your wellbeing business stand out in an increasingly crowded digital marketplace. We will cover these aspects in the next chapter but first let us look at other avenues.

Giving talks and demonstrations

When I first began working as a reflexologist I gave many talks to local interest groups. Although daunting at first, it quickly became one of my most effective marketing tools. More often than not I gained at least one new client with each talk that I gave. Giving a talk will allow you to educate and engage with your local community and will enable you to show the benefits of what you have to offer as well as your passion and knowledge for your wellbeing subject.

There are many groups in your local community who are looking for interesting passionate speakers; the first place to start to find them is with an internet search. In my experience if you give one or two talks you will then start to be noticed by other groups and get invitations to speak at these.

My first talk was to my local women's group. I started by giving a 20-minute talk about the history and benefits of reflexology then followed it with a physical demonstration pointing out the reflexes as I went, then finishing with a questions and answers.

Within my first two years I did not just speak to local women's groups, I spoke at networking events and local businesses including tax office employees. Many businesses provide wellbeing events for their employees and are always looking for local wellbeing professionals to attend these.

Although many interest groups and businesses are unable to pay you to give these talks; more often than not they are prepared to pay your travel expenses. As I have already said speaking proved to not just be a good way of gaining new clients it also helped me to hone my marketing message, build my credibility and confidence.

Printed leaflets/flyers

When I trained as a reflexologist in 2000 the only piece of advice about marketing I was given was how to create a leaflet to advertise my reflexology service. In today's digital world it is easy to forget about the power of printed materials such as leaflets, flyers and business cards. A well-designed thought provoking leaflet/flyer can be a low cost and effective way to advertise your therapy/class.

Tips for creating a leaflet or flyer

- Remember the old saying 'less is more'. Do not be tempted to fill every corner of your leaflet with lots of text; people have a tendency to scan leaflets rather than read all of the text.

- Use high quality images, whether you use your own images or copy write free stock photographs from the internet, ensure they are of a high enough quality to be printed. A good quality images showcases the quality of your work.

- Your titles should grab your client's attention

- There are many free online platforms to help you create a professional looking leaflet.

Here are some suggestions about what to include in your leaflet, the history of your therapy is not necessary:

- About your business

- Include your business mission statement

- Services

- Highlight your services, discuss the benefits, and a little of the interesting or unique facts about them.

- Qualifications

- Include your qualifications, insurance and any membership bodies you belong to.

- About you

- A short paragraph about yourself and why you work in wellbeing

- Testimonials

- Including 2 or 3 genuine testimonials.

- Contact details

- Including your website and any social media links, as well as where you practice or teach from.

- Price

- Not everyone agrees about whether your prices should be included or not. There are arguments on both sides.

When designing your leaflet try to keep your paragraphs and sentences short; remembering the adage 'less is more'. I would advise you to start, small placing leaflets in local shops and cafes.

Content marketing

Content marketing is about creating and sharing interesting and helpful, free content that resonates with your ideal client. Marketing in this way is a long-term strategy designed to help you build relationships with potential clients. Good content does not just demonstrate your skills; it also shows that you care about their wellbeing, it helps clients to get a sense of who you are, what you believe and your trustworthiness, so, when they need your services they will know just where to come.

There are a lot of opportunities to content market; for example, videos, blogs for your own website and others, vlogs, e-books, podcasts, newsletters and social media. It does not all have to be online. You may want to write an article for a local magazine or a press release to a journalist.

The vast amount of choice can be a little overwhelming. I suggest you pick two or three and concentrate on doing those well. If your ideal client is someone who loves watching videos then it would make sense to choose video making as one of your options. Equally if the idea of writing blog posts seems overwhelming and time consuming to you it is probably best to avoid this option - at least in the beginning.

Deciding what to post, write or vlog about can be very daunting. Start by thinking what is it that your ideal client wants to know. What can you tell them today that will help them with their wellbeing?

A year or so ago I created a short video entitled 'Do you feel guilty about charging for your wellbeing services?' This particular video has had more views than any other video I have created; the reason being is because I have tried to provide answers to a common problem wellbeing professionals struggle with.

If you are not sure what to include in your content marketing then think back to your own story, the reasons why you decided to work in wellbeing. Your mission statement will also help you to create content that is helpful, authentic and heartfelt.

Do not worry if you are struggling to get started. I suggest you look at some of the content produced by people you admire and look up to. What is it that attracted you to read or listen to something they have created in the first place? I am not suggesting you copy or plagiarise their work, just pay attention to what it is that works for them. Content does not have to be perfect or polished, it does however, have to stand out from the competition, you do have to be a little brave and put yourself out there. We are all attracted to someone who we feel shows passion and authenticity.

Traditional print advertising

Not so long ago placing an advert in a local newspaper was a 'must have' for a local business. A local paper functioned like a directory of local services. Now fewer businesses are using this method of advertising, however, I know of several therapists and teachers who still use this method and find it generates them new clients.

If you decide to use print advertising it is important to remember that the vast majority of people flick through magazines, they do not read every line. With this in mind, your design needs to be simple and bold with an attention-grabbing headline; you have approximately 2 seconds to attract a person's attention. Resist the temptation to cram in a lot of unnecessary detail. The purpose of your advert it to tempt potential clients to find out more about you.

Before placing your advert, you need to ask a few questions about the magazine.

- How many people does their magazine reach? It is not uncommon for a magazine to tell you a figure for example 10,000 which sounds fantastic but be aware that 2,000 of those may be delivered to local business that just put them straight into a recycling bin or leave them on a coffee table where they never get opened.

- In what areas is the magazine delivered?

- What kind of readers does the magazine attract?

By asking these questions you are checking whether or not the publication delivers to your ideal client.

If you decide to place magazine adverts, I would suggest that you budget for at least three months' worth of advertising; your potential clients need to see you are going to stay around and can trust you. It is unusual for a client to decide to use your services the first time they see your advert.

Business Cards

There is no doubt that business cards are not used as much today as they were even 5 years ago, now many people are swapping information digitally. I believe that business cards still have a place in today's digital world.

There are so many opportunities to network and connect with like-minded people. I have given my business card to people, in coffee shops or when I have been waiting for my children at their swimming lessons. One of my wellbeing business friends once gave her business card to the cashier at Ikea when she was buying glasses. She was running a yoga event; the subject came up and the cashier was interested in coming along. You just never know when the opportunity arises.

A memorable business card does more than just share your contact details it also gives the receiver a first impression of who you are and what your brand stands for. Whether you decide to design your own business card or pay a designer to do it for you, it is worth taking the time to produce a business card design that accurately represents what your business stands for.

Media Coverage

If you want to get media coverage for your wellbeing business a press release is a good way to do this. A press release is a clearly written communication telling journalists and bloggers about your story.

A press release should have a headline that is attention grabbing; remember that journalists are busy people you will only have a limited amount of time to get them interested. When you are writing your press release, try to answer the following questions.

- **Who?** Is this about; you or your clients.

- **What?** Is the story.

- **Why?** Do people need to know about this

- **Where?** Is it taking place (if this is relevant).

- **When?** Is it happening (if this is relevant).

- **How?** Did this come about.

The key to success with a press release is persistence, it may just be a matter of timing; your press release may just arrive on a journalist's desk when they are looking for a story just like yours.

If you are not convinced of the effectiveness of media coverage for your wellbeing business let me give you an example. In 2014 Philip Humphreys a craniosacral therapist who works at my Clinic was featured in the Daily Mail newspaper for his work with babies. Although this did not come about directly through a press release the article has had a profound effect on his business even today. The article was written in 2014 but is still circulating the internet now and is regularly found by parents looking for help with their babies.

Appearances on radio and local television

A few years ago, I had a regular slot on local radio station. Apart from being great fun it was a good way to raise my clinic profile. I loved nothing more than talking to people about the benefits of wellbeing.

If this appeals to you, it is easier than you would think to get yourself on local radio and television. Simply contacting them through their e-mail or social media may be enough. They are always looking for interesting people to feature.

TAKE ACTION

At this stage, I want you to start thinking about the usefulness of different marketing methods. The questions and tasks below are designed to get you thinking creatively.

- Identify some local interest group you could give a talk to about your wellbeing business.

- Find three leaflets that advertise the same treatment/class you offer. Of the three, which one attracts you and why? Is it the visuals, the words etc.

- Take some time to really look at the blogs, pod casts or videos you personally follow. It does not have to be in your industry; sometimes it is helpful to look outside of our industry and look at how they do things elsewhere - it is a great way to spark creativity. Why do you follow them? Do they tell you what to do next?

- Identify publications in your area and contact them to find out how much they charge to advertise.

- Write a list of the publications you would like to appear in locally and nationally.

Trust in yourself,
you are on the
right path.

CHAPTER TEN

YOUR WELLBEING BUSINESS AND THE INTERNET

In today's world, it has never been easier to reach so many people; the internet has made this possible. There are lots of opportunities to network and promote yourself online. 10 years ago, my marketing budget was a lot bigger than it is now; I no longer spend a large sum of money on magazine advertising and yellow pages adverts. However, on the internet it is easy to get lost in the crowd of other wellbeing business owners trying to do the same thing.

In this chapter, we will look at websites and social media. Not as a manual on how to set up a website or all the ins and outs of social media, but it is designed to show you all the information you need to think about when creating your online sales tools.

Some of the options will require a financial investment others will be free but all will require an investment of your time. By the end of this chapter you will be able to make informed choices about your online marketing mix.

Website

Nowadays, it is nearly impossible to have a business without a website. Clients use the internet like we used to use the yellow pages or local paper. In the UK, 9 out of 10 adults use the internet.

A good website is an invaluable tool, a digital shop window for your clients. It is the place where your clients find out if you have the solution to their problems. However, I often go on to wellbeing business websites and struggle to find the information I want. You have around 60 secs to gets someone's attention before they click off and on to the next website.

This is not long, so what do your clients need to see?

Tips to create a trustworthy website

- If you decide to build your own website. There are many website building platforms that are intuitive and easy to use as well as being very reasonably priced. If you cannot face building your own website, you can use a professional website designer. Take the time to shop around with either option; prices and quality vary greatly.

- Taking the time to look at other company's websites, not necessarily only in the wellbeing industry, will help you see where clients expect to see key elements, such as logo, headers and footers, contact information and navigation bars. As you only have 60 seconds to gain someone's attention make it easy for clients to find the information they need.

- As a local business, it is essential that your clients can find exactly where you are, do not just put your location in your footer. Make sure it is in the banner on the home page or any page that a client is likely to come to first. One of the first things a client is going to want to know when they are looking for a service is where it is located.

- Ensure your website expresses clearly what you do. If you are an aromatherapist then say it; make this a priority on your home page I have read a lot of websites that do not make it clear what they are selling until you are half way down the home page - this is too late.

- When you write your website copy keep in mind your ideal client profile from chapter 6 - imagine you are writing for them. Avoid writing unnecessary information, remember your clients are looking to see if you can provide them with the help they want and need. Many people only scan websites, so resist the temptation to put in unnecessary sentences and jargon. You need to create a balance between information and interest.

- Resist the temptation to use the 'we' word if you work on your own. You are fooling no one by using the word 'we' it does not make you look bigger or more established than you are. It is much more genuine to fill your website with your own personality and authenticity; this creates connection and trust with your clients.

- Your website needs to be visually enticing. You do not have to have a budget for professional pictures and logos there are many stock photo and logo websites where you can get pictures and logos at very reasonable prices or free. Ensure that you have a good clear picture of yourself and remember it does not need to be professionally taken. A picture of you will help clients to feel an emotional connection with you.

- Make sure that your website is optimised for search engines. You can get a lot of tips on how to do this by searching "search engine optimisation" or SEO into google. You can do a lot of search engine optimisation yourself without outsourcing to another company.

- Essentially SEO is about creating unique, interesting and relevant content for your readers. Take time to think about the words and terms your prospective clients are likely to type into a search engine. For example, if your client wants to book a hot stone massage, they are likely to type in the words hot stone massage followed by the area they want it to be in. Ensure that these words are found in your copy, heading and web address. Search engines are going to provide what they

FROM CLIENT TO CLINIC OWNER

consider to be the most relevant websites in response to what the user types in to the search engine.

- Including testimonials build trust. Potential clients want to know about the experiences existing clients have already had.

As with all marketing tools you need to know if your website is working for you. Many website platforms will also include some sort of analytics or alternatively Google offer some free analytics tool. This provides you with comprehensive information about how many people are using your website, what key words they are using and how long they are staying on your website.

TAKE ACTION

_____

A useful exercise, either before writing your own website or testing your existing one, is to look at other wellbeing business websites as though you are a potential client.

Pick five websites that offer similar services to you. Now imagine you are looking to book a therapy or class.

- Do these websites provide the information you need to make a decision?
- How easy are they to navigate?
- How many clicks do you have to make before you book?

Whether you decide to take the plunge and build your own website or employ the services of a website builder, you now have a good idea of what should be included.

Social Media

The subject of social media is a book in itself and I will be the first to admit I am not a social media expert. However, over 70% of internet owners have some sort of social media presence. Social media is about connecting and listening to your audience. Your existing and future clients want to see your human side, your authentic voice, the passion you have for wellbeing.

A few years ago, there was a general sense that you needed to be on every social media platform that existed. I found this tiresome and overwhelming. I ended up with a lot of my content being duplicated or I would forget to post on one of them. So, I decided to concentrate my efforts on just one social media platform, Facebook. Personally, I find this the easiest to use, it suits my personal style I like Facebook's ability to share more content than Twitter and I prefer it to the more formal style of LinkedIn.

Building your audience on social media is a learning curve; it takes time and practice so be prepared to try different post styles, post at different times of the day and post regularly.

Tips for making the most of social media

- As I have said I choose Facebook as my main social media marketing. The main reason being is that this is where most of my prospective clients are, as well as being the platform that resonates the most with me personally. However, if your clients are on Twitter, Pinterest, Snapchat, Instagram, LinkedIn or Google plus then pick one or as many as you can effectively handle.

- Whichever social media platforms you decide to use it is important to be clear about your purpose and aim. I use Facebook to attract and engage with my clients from here I want to drive them to my website and turn them into paying clients.

- Knowing who your clients are will make it easier for you to find them and tell your story in a way that resonates with them. This is the place to use your ideal client profile from chapter 6.

- When you are thinking about content for your social media posts, do not think about what you want to tell them but think about what they want to know. For example, if you are an acupuncturist many clients want to know if the needles hurt. You could do a post dispelling the myths surrounding acupuncture.

- Always be authentic and true to yourself. This will help you to come across as human and helpful.

- Post about the value you offer, what you offer for clients and why. Use your mission statement. If you are a reflexologist whose aim is to help women move through the menopause in the most natural way possible then say so.

- If you want people to engage with your social media posts, make sure you reciprocate, engage and start conversations with them.

- Do not bombard people with sales posts. Social media is the place to talk about your lifestyle as an individual. Clients want to know who you are as a person, what you are passionate about. However, that being said, put your boundaries in place – you do not need to share everything about yourself and your life, just what is relevant to your wellbeing business.

Advertising online

I would encourage you to set aside some time to start to understand how paid internet advertising works if you get it right it can be a very cost-effective means of gaining new clients; get it wrong and you can easily spend a lot of money with little or no success. Pay per click advertising and social media advertising are two popular ways wellbeing business owners can find new clients.

Pay per click advertising - is generally run by search engines. You pay when someone clicks on your advert. For example, one of your clients may be looking for an Indian Head Massage near where they live, they type into the search engine what they are looking for in the area they want it. The search engine then filters the results based on the relevance of your advert to the client's search; if your advert shows and the client clicks on your advert or link you will then be charged.

The benefits of this method of advertising is you can put a lot of focus on to the 'key words' your clients might use i.e. 'Indian Head Massage' and the area you are located. You can create adverts that will be specifically targeted at those people who will be interested in what you have to offer.

Social media advertising – once you have got used to running your social media accounts in a way that works for you and your client you may decide you want to take it further and have a go at advertising with them. As with pay per click advertising you can set a budget then create audiences based around your ideal client, age, location, gender, likes and dislikes.

I use both these methods of online advertising; it is a good way to get your wellbeing business in front of your ideal client. It does, however, take time to learn how to advertise effectively online. I suggest starting with a small budget and measure the results with the analytical tools online companies provide.

What do you need to do to make real change? It's simple; care about other people.

CHAPTER ELEVEN

NETWORKING

Networking, whether on- or off-line, is a skill that every wellbeing business owner is going to have to learn especially in the early days of your wellbeing business. You actively have to share information about you and your business; your clients need to know who you are and what you have to offer them.

A good place to start is with your friends and acquaintances. But I do not suggest you spend hours boring you friends about your wellbeing business or trying to strong arm them into having a treatment or come along to a class, you will quickly loose friends, this way.

However, friends will be interested in supporting you. Beginning to talk with them about what you do will help you hone your voice, message and confidence. Networking is not just about finding new business. I have found many useful suppliers, contacts and collaborations through casual conversations with acquaintances often in the most unlikely places.

Having said this, you cannot just rely on your existing friends and contacts to help you grow your wellbeing business; you will also have to sometimes put yourself in unfamiliar situations. If you are someone who is very confident or who is used to networking, maybe from a previous job, then you may find this easy once you have honed your message.

However, for a lot of wellbeing business owners networking will be a new experience and you may find the idea of talking about yourself and your wellbeing business terrifying.

When I first started networking as a new therapist the world of networking was indeed a strange and scary place. Networking was about having a bacon sandwich with a bunch of middle aged business men. We had to stand up and do a one minute presentation about our business in a windowless hotel conference room. An enlightening experience for a shy, female, vegetarian, introvert with a passion for wellbeing. Thankfully today there are many more exciting opportunities to meet and connect with like-minded people.

However, I am thankful for those early days of networking. I met some amazing business people who helped me grow my business. I learnt a lot about myself and how to present my business in an effective way. I learnt how to be creative with my one minute presentations -you have to be if you want to keep the attention of a group of people who have listened to 10 presentations already and are really thinking about their breakfast. The result being I got over my fear of public speaking.

Thankfully over the years, I have developed in my understanding of networking and have developed a much better way of networking that suits me and my needs.

Now, you appreciate that you need to network to build your business but to what purpose? Networking helps you tap into your local community and build relationships. These relationships will help you gain:

- New business for your therapy or class.

- Introductions to people who can help you build your knowledge.

- Word of mouth recommendations for suppliers for your business.

- Potential partners or collaborators.

- Inspiration and encouragement.

The more you connect and network the more events you will be asked to attend and the wider your network and reach.

By putting yourself out into the community you will find people who want to help you grow your wellbeing business and will help put you in touch with others who can do the same.

You will also want to help other businesses grow their business. As a wellbeing clinic owner, I am always interested in other wellbeing businesses and if I can help I will, my clinic website has a blog I am always looking for new and interesting content. If a wellbeing business is offering a service or product that I don't have in my clinic I invite them to write a blog for us that I then share on our social media. This gives them some added exposure and I gain fresh content for my readers. The result is a collaboration that benefits both of our businesses.

If the idea of networking still sounds terrifying let me share some of the tips I have learnt over the years. Although I networked a lot in the early days of my business I was so focused on building, learning and getting over my fears that I did not necessarily approach the process in the most mindful of ways I learnt a lot but was very stressed.

As the years went by, my business grew and I began to get fed up with the constant round of networking meetings I was exhausted and felt emotionally drained with what I thought was a lack of genuine and authentic connection.

This was around the time that social media was beginning to take off I needed a break from face to face networking and the rise social media networking allowed me to do this. I was able to take the time to work on some personal development, I realised that I actually have a lot of introverted tendencies.

Although I can put myself out there in networking situations, I then need a lot of time on my own to recover and regroup. I prefer smaller more intimate groups or coffee dates where I can make authentic connections. I like to be fully present when talking to someone not looking over their shoulder for the next person I want talk to or thinking about my dinner. I prefer to ask questions and listen to the other persons responses I have learnt more and made much deeper connections this way.

These realisations reframed networking for me. I am now more discerning about the amount of networking I attended. Instead of feeling as though I need to connect with everyone in a room I like to connect authentically with a smaller amount of people.

TAKE ACTION

If you are new to networking I want to challenge you attend a local networking group. Talk to one or two people in the room. Ask questions about their business, find out how they got started in their business and ask them how you might be able to help. These questions will open up the conversation.

Putting yourself and your business out in the world is a little scary so start small. What seems scary now will become easier very quickly and you never know you may just make a friend that helps you gain more business.

Your clients are partners in your wellbeing business, love and amaze them.

CHAPTER TWELVE

LOVE AND AMAZE YOUR CLIENTS

So often the focus for marketing is about gaining new clients. We spend a lot of time, money and energy trying to get new clients. However, to grow a sustainable wellbeing business you need to retain your existing clients. If you look after and reward your existing clients they will return time and time again, refer new clients to you, and write you testimonials.

As a new reflexologist, back in 2001 it was not until I learnt how to help my clients rebook that my wellbeing business began to be grow. Once I learned how to do this I gained not just a profitable practice for myself but a greater sense of satisfaction seeing my clients get the results they wanted because they were choosing to return for more treatment.

Providing you client with the best treatment or class you can offer is only part of the story. Even though therapists and teachers know that it benefits their clients to return for a course of treatment or attend regular classes many therapists and teachers struggle to rebook their clients.

For new wellbeing business owners, the process of rebooking can often feel awkward and a little to salesy. Let us look at it another way. Yes, you need to get your clients to rebook but rather than viewing it as you trying to gain another sale; look at it as if you are educating your clients about the benefits and value they will achieve by returning for regular sessions.

So, how do we do this? The process of rebooking your clients starts from the moment you fill in their intake form. This is when you learn about their health goals, what is it they want to achieve by coming to see you. By really listening to what it is you client wants to achieve you can educate them about the benefits of regular treatment.

If your client feels as though you have really listened and heard them they are more likely to rebook, you are starting to develop a relationship based on trust. This is a good foundation for helping you clients achieve their health goals.

Even though you have shown your client the value and benefits you can offer them it is still essential that you offer to book their next appointment whilst they are paying. Remember that once they step out of your door they will be bombarded by life and all of its responsibilities. Booking their next appointment will quickly move down the priority list of everything else they have to do.

It is important to be specific with your recommendations if you feel they should come and see you once a week for six weeks to really see the benefits of your treatment then this is what you should recommend. They are after all paying for your advice, as well as your services.

Over the years I have witnessed many therapists be vague about when a client should return for fear of being too pushy. Statements such as, "see how you get on" or "it's up to you" leaves the client confused and unsure what to do for the best. The result more often than not is that they leave without making a booking, never to return.

Remember, they felt confident enough to book a therapy or attend your class, now they need your opinion and advice as to when to return and follow up with you.

Instead of being vague try saying statements such as, "would you like to book an appointment for next week" or "I have availability the same time next week."

TAKE ACTION

I want you to think of a time you had a therapy appointment. Think about how the therapist talked to you after the treatment. Did they offer you advice about when to come back and after care? Did they offer to re-book you after the appointment? How did this make you feel? Did you feel safe and secure in the knowledge that they were the expert and you were glad they offered their advice? Or did you feel sold to?

Now think of a situation where you had the most amazing treatment but no advice was offered about when to come back.

- Did you want to know but didn't dare ask?
- Did you walk away thinking, wow that was amazing I must go back?
- Did you go back?
- Would you have preferred them to advise you or not?

As we have seen helping your clients rebook with you is not about being salesy it is about offering them the advice they have paid for. Ultimately it is up to the client whether they decide to return to you or not, your job is to make it as easy as possible for them.

Testimonials

> Testimonial: "something given or done as an expression of esteem, admiration, or gratitude."
>
> Dictionary definition

Do not underestimate the power of a testimonial to increase your business especially in today's internet world. Good testimonials can dramatically increase your business; clients are more likely to buy from a business that has good, genuine client testimonials. A testimonial demonstrates your expertise and credibility. It also demonstrates the trust your existing clients have for you. These are all qualities a prospective client will be looking for in a therapist or teacher. Your marketing shows clients what you can do for them; a testimonial proves that you can deliver on what you are saying.

Have you ever bought something because a friend recommended it? Maybe you tried a restaurant because a friend loved it or watched a film because someone mentioned how good it was. These are verbal testimonials. Happy clients spread the word about your wellbeing business.

We know that testimonials are important so how do we gather them? You cannot wait around hoping that your clients will write them without you mentioning it.

The most effective way to gather testimonials is by asking for them face to face. If your client has had a good experience with you, achieved a health goal they had, then ask if they would like to leave you a testimonial and tell them where you would like them to write it. Suggest e-mailing them a link to where you would like them to leave the testimonial i.e. Facebook, Google plus or Yell. Remember writing testimonials is not easy it can be a good idea to include an example of the sort of testimonial you would like within the same e-mail. Make the experience as easy as possible for them.

Example testimonial:

> "I had an amazing aromatherapy massage today with
> _____, really great.... I almost fell asleep I was so
> relaxed! Totally recommend it."

I know it can feel a little embarrassing and awkward to ask for a testimonial, but remember that most people want to help you grow your business. Ensure that you do not just use your testimonials on your social media. Incorporate them into your website as well and make it easy for your prospective clients to find and read them.

TAKE ACTION

——

Challenge yourself to get three testimonials. Talk to your clients and ask them to write a short testimonial for you.

Customer service

I love good customer service it makes me feel special. It makes me happy that I chose to spend my money in the place where I get good customer service.

I love my local coffee shop, they always remember my name and my coffee order.

One of the simplest ways to retain your clients is to provide amazing customer service. The little things are what make the big difference and will keep your clients coming back time and time again.

Tips for providing excellent customer service

- Take the time to remember your clients name. Although this may seem obvious I have had the experience more than once of returning for a therapy session where the therapist clearly couldn't remember my name.

- Smile when you greet your client. A genuine smile helps a client to relax and get over any fears they may have about coming for treatment, a smile helps to build trust and make them feel good about themselves and their decision to spend money with you.

- Respond promptly to a client's enquiry there is nothing more off putting than waiting too long before getting a response to an e-mail or phone message.

- Add value to their experience with you. A little extra can go a long way to impressing your clients. For example, if you are a massage therapist you could provide a basket or clothes hangers for your client to put their clothes on rather than just putting them on a chair.

- Keep your promises. If you say you are going to e-mail your client a list of exercises or a link to an amazing meditation app make sure that you follow through.

- Reward clients who refer you knew clients. It may be as simple as a thank you card or an aromatherapy oil.

- Reward loyalty. At my own clinic, we offer a loyalty card over the years this have proved to be very successful. However, make sure you do your sums and check you can afford the discount you are offering.

- Remembering a client's birthday with a card or e-mail you may want to include a gift of a treatment or class.

- Deal with any clients quickly and promptly.

Remember good customer service really does make a difference.

Surround yourself with people who believe in what you are doing.

CHAPTER THIRTEEN

FINDING SUPPORT, SELF-CARE AND HEALTHY BOUNDARIES

I remember when I first started working as a reflexologist and trying to explain to my gran what I did for a living. I really struggled to explain reflexology to her, I think she thought I was just rubbing people's feet for a living. I realised very quickly that it is really difficult to explain to people your desire to work for yourself and how challenging it can be at times.

The self-employment journey can be a lonely one, there are no colleagues to chat to when you are stuck on a problem or feeling a lack of motivation.

It is really important that you get support, from business friends, mentors or coaches. Surround yourself with as many people as possible who understand the journey you are on.

The benefit of business friends is that you do not have to explain the journey to them. Occasionally a group of my wellbeing business friends meet for dinner or go out for a drink. We created a space for ourselves where we could vent and laugh about all the craziness that is self-employment. Although we are in an informal setting we are able to offer encouragement to each other, celebrate the successes and help with issues.

Your business friends do not have to be in the same industry as you; some of my best advice and support has come from friends who work in very different industry sectors to me.

There are many supportive closed networking groups online that can offer you support and guidance around self-employment.

However, I would recommend that you find yourself a mentor or coach. They may be someone you pay and enter into a formal relationship with or are a therapist, wellbeing teacher, who has already built a business the next size up from yours. Just remember the role of a mentor and coach is to facilitate you to grow your wellbeing business, not do it for you. Bearing that in mind make sure you have an idea of what you want help with.

My coaches and mentors have not only acted as a sounding board for my ideas they have made me accountable for my decisions. Like most entrepreneurs I am really good at seeing the big vision for my business however, at times I can struggle with the details. Working with coaches has helped me pay attention to these areas of my businesses and kept me moving forward.

TAKE ACTION

———

Write a list of those business people who you want to be surrounded with. Then make it happen - arrange a night out. Investigate a coach or mentor who could bring value to your business.

It is not lost on me that I am writing a chapter about self-care for people who work in wellbeing. Self-care and setting healthy boundaries around your work can be a challenge when you are full of passion for what you do.

You have to balance classes/practice alongside working on your business with all your other commitments, never mind finding sometime for yourself.

In the early days, you may be happy to spend every waking hour working and thinking about your business. Fast forward five years, if you do not take some time for yourself there is a high risk you will burn out and fall out of love with what you do.

I am not going to tell you what you should do to care of yourself; after all I am guessing you are an expert in that. I am going to provide you with some tips on how and where you can reduce stress in your business.

Tips to reduce the stress and set boundaries for yourself

- The first few years of business can be especially hard because you have no bench mark as to the natural ebb and flow of your business; certain times of the year you will be busier than others. This lack of knowledge can create a lot of stress. You may have been building nicely then you have a bad month you start to doubt everything you are doing. Ensure that you keep up to date records month on month as to how your business is growing. By doing this you will have a reference point to look back on. Some months are naturally better than others. The slower months are for cultivating new projects and planning.

- We all have different energy levels, recognise and honour this. Do not fall into the trap of comparing the amount of work you are doing with what you perceive someone else to be doing. I do not have the same energy that I had in my thirties however, these days I am much more productive.

- When you take a holiday resist the temptation to check your messages, there is very little that cannot wait for a few days.

- Set boundaries around answering e-mails and phone calls. Yes, you do need to reply promptly to enquiries but as long as you have messages on your phone etc. that say when you will respond. Your customers will honour and respect this

- If you draw energy from sending lots of time on your own then make the time; go for a walk, meditate, do yoga, whatever it is that you need to do. Alternatively, if you draw your energy from being surrounded by your friends then make a date with them and have some fun.

- If you need a job on the side to keep the money flowing in whilst you grow your wellbeing business then do it. Good things take time to grow; your clients will not benefit from your talents if you have to stop because you cannot afford to live.

I love social media both personally and for my business however, I have found it is vital to set myself boundaries around how I use it. Otherwise I can find myself spending hours on social media constantly checking for updates, who has liked or who has commented on my business posts. Although I can get a lot of inspiration from following and reading peoples posts on social media, it can equally work the other way. I can quickly become overwhelmed with information and fall into the trap of comparisons.

If I am not careful I can lose my creativity and paralyse myself into doing nothing or worrying that other business people are doing better than me, that I am not being spiritual enough, not meditating or practicing enough yoga. Social media is an amazing tool that allows you to connect and hone your message like never before. But recognise that it is not a substitute for connecting with people in person.

Being self- employed and setting boundaries around your work is very different from being employed. You have to master the art of self-discipline at times you will have to work hard and take the opportunities that come your way. That is ok because self-employment is not a 9-5 job. You do however, have to balance work with time for yourself and make sure that you are fully present with those around you when you are with them.

A plan gives your dreams life.

CHAPTER FOURTEEN

DO YOU NEED A BUSINESS PLAN?

Writing a business plan for your wellbeing business is something that most therapists and teachers feel they should do. They may have been told by other 'business people' that it is essential to write a business plan to be successful, or alternatively they may have heard some entrepreneurs say they have never used a business plan.

It is not surprising that you may then be confused as to whether you need a business plan or not. In this chapter I am going to share my experience of business plans and why I believe it is helpful to have a plan – whatever you want to call it.

Do you need growth forecasts and three-year plans to make your wellbeing business a success? Probably not. Do you need a basic idea of your costs and your break-even point? Yes, it would be unwise not to do this.

I understand the idea of writing a huge document and spending a lot of time working on it can feel overwhelming, not to mention annoying. I would much rather be working on growing my business and getting my wellbeing message out to my clients. Like most business people I find it much easier and more exciting to see the big business picture rather than get caught up into too much detail. Sometimes I feel as though this level of detail dulls my intuition and creativity.

But, and there is big but…. nearly half of all businesses in the United Kingdom fail in their first year. I would argue a plan of some description can help you to avoid becoming one of those statistics.

When I wanted to buy the Wellbeing Clinic I needed to raise capital, so I had to create a business plan for the bank. It was a huge document full of cash flow forecasts, 3 year plans and rambling explanations of my skills and how I was going to run and grow the Wellbeing Clinic. It took at least 2 months to complete and once it was finished and handed to the bank. It served its purpose and helped me to raise the capital I needed to buy and open the Wellbeing Clinic. However, it did little else.

I still have this business plan, it is kept in a filing cabinet in my office and has never been opened again in over 15 years, I have not used it to help me steer the business in any way, it was too overwhelming, it was not written in a language that I found helpful.

The one thing I do know is that the next 3 business years of the Wellbeing Clinic were nothing like what my business plan predicted.

In the intervening years, I learnt a lot about myself and how to run a heartfelt business in line with my own personal values.

Do I think there is still value in writing a business plan? Absolutely, but it should be no longer than a couple of pages and written in a style that works for your business. Your plan should support you to align your personal and business values with your business goals and objectives. Whether you are a therapist working on your own or are planning to open a yoga studio with other therapists and teachers a heartfelt useable business plan will help you move forward and allow you to use your healing skill to maximum effect.

If I knew what I know now I would have achieved my goals much more quickly and saved myself a lot of money and stress. I would have developed a heartfelt plan not necessarily a traditional "business plan".

If you have done the exercises in the book you should have all the information you need to write a short usable plan for yourself.

Journeying
through life in the
most authentic way
I can; knowledge
seeker, client,
holistic therapist,
clinic owner.

CHAPTER FIFTEEN

IT'S ALL A JOURNEY

Congratulations you have come this far you are working really hard to make your wellbeing business a success. You should be really proud of yourself.

Creating your dream wellbeing business will push you to do things you have never done before and search inside yourself in ways that you have never imagined. I know this has been my experience. My business journey has taken me to places I would never imagine I could go. I would never have thought myself capable of writing a book.

I have discovered that I am very persistent. This is definitely a quality that business owners need to develop. Even if you have worked through all of this book and you have gained clarity about your mission, you are marketing to your ideal clients and have a clear plan with achievable goals, sometimes progress can feel frustratingly slow.

At times throughout my wellbeing career there have been times when I have questioned and doubted myself especially in the early days of owning my clinic. There were times when I was tempted to quit and get a "proper job".

Especially when I could see my friends setting up their own businesses that appeared to be more successful than mine or friends that were being promoted within their jobs and becoming financially secure.

Despite my worries and doubts, underneath it all I knew that I was on the right path - wellbeing was my future. I needed to keep going and be persistent; it takes time for clients to find you and trust that you are going to stick around.

Trust me when I say every business owner has doubts and experiences problems from time to time. It is all part of the journey.

The tough times are there to help us fine tune our message and processes. When you are feeling unsure look, listen and feel into what it is you need to learn. In my experience, the same problems will keep appearing in different forms until it has shown you what you need to change.

At times like this I have seen therapists and teachers have a minor panic, they doubt their ability to fill their practices or class so they add in another therapy a different class or start to sell products. I encourage you to focus on one thing at a time and learn to make that work before you add in another service or product you need to sell.

Be persistent and surround yourself with people who understand that you are on a journey.

A FINAL WORD

You are working hard to create a wellbeing business you love. I hope this book has helped you to realise that it is possible to create a business that helps lots of people and provides you with a living.

It is my genuine wish that you succeed in your practice; the more of us that do the more people benefit from the wonderful world of holistic health.

Working as a therapist or teacher can at times feel lonely. I hope this book helps you to feel supported as you journey along. I hope that if you were feeling stuck and uninspired you are now ready to look at your business anew.

Yes, there are lots of holistic therapists, mindfulness and yoga teachers out there but I hope this book has shown you that by taking the time to learn who you are in your business and where your unique skills lie you are more than equipped to find the clients you are supposed to be working with.

I encourage you to keep this book to hand and revisit it from time to time. It is meant as a handy guide to use when you need. The exercises can be repeated as many times as you like. As you move through your business life, you will grow and change and so will your business - the exercises will help you embrace these changes.

With gratitude,

Helen

ABOUT THE AUTHOR

Helen has a passion for all aspects of wellbeing and a lifelong passion for learning.

She has created three businesses dedicated to counselling, coaching and alternative health.

Her curiosity for business started as a child helping her mother sell Christmas crackers, firstly at craft fairs and then trade fairs.

After university and several failed attempts at different jobs and careers she realised she literally had no idea what she wanted to do.

Whilst struggling to conceive her first child, Helen stumbled upon the world of complementary health and there found her passion, first as a therapist then as a clinic owner.

Helen believes success is having the courage to listen to our heart and desires, to not become stuck by our fears. Being true to ourselves we can bring our values and passions to the world serving the customers we are meant to serve.

38474830R00105

Printed in Poland
by Amazon Fulfillment
Poland Sp. z o.o., Wrocław